CONTENTS

INTRODUCTION

Welcome Message

Welcome to **"Vigor & Vitality: Quick and Easy Recipes for Men's Sexual Health"**! This book is your guide to enhancing your sexual health through delicious and nutritious recipes. Whether you're looking to boost your libido, improve stamina, or maintain overall reproductive health, the right foods can make a significant difference. Our recipes are designed to be quick, easy, and packed with ingredients that support your sexual health and well-being.

Overview of the Book's Purpose

The purpose of this book is to promote men's sexual health through nutrition. Sexual health is an essential aspect of overall well-being, and what you eat plays a crucial role in maintaining and enhancing it. By incorporating certain foods into your diet, you can improve blood flow, hormone levels, and energy, all of which are vital for a healthy sex life. This book provides a variety of recipes that are not only easy to prepare but also rich in nutrients known to support sexual health.

Importance of a Balanced Diet in Maintaining Sexual Health

A balanced diet is the foundation of good health, including sexual health. The right combination of nutrients can help maintain healthy hormone levels, improve blood circulation, and provide the energy needed for a fulfilling sex life. Conversely, a poor diet can lead to problems such as reduced libido, erectile dysfunction, and other health issues that affect sexual performance. By focusing on a diet rich in vitamins, minerals, and other essential nutrients, you can enhance your sexual health and overall well-being.

Types of Food That Can Help

Fruits and Vegetables

Bananas: Bananas are rich in potassium and vitamin B6, which help increase energy levels and testosterone production. They also contain bromelain, an enzyme that can help boost libido.

Watermelon: Watermelon contains citrulline, an amino acid that can help relax blood vessels and improve blood flow, similar to how certain medications work to treat erectile dysfunction.

Avocados: Avocados are high in vitamin E, which enhances sperm quality, and potassium, which boosts libido. They also contain healthy fats that support hormone production.

Spinach: Spinach is packed with magnesium, which helps dilate blood vessels, improving blood flow to the genitals. It's also a great source of folate, which is essential for overall sexual health.

Nuts and Seeds

Almonds: Almonds are rich in zinc, selenium, and vitamin E, which can enhance libido and sexual health. They also provide healthy fats and protein for sustained energy.

Walnuts: Walnuts are high in omega-3 fatty acids, which improve blood flow and enhance sperm quality. They also contain antioxidants that support overall health.

Pumpkin Seeds: Pumpkin seeds are high in zinc, which is crucial for testosterone production and sperm health. They also provide magnesium and healthy fats.

Lean Proteins

Salmon: Salmon is high in omega-3 fatty acids, which improve cardiovascular health and blood flow. It also provides protein and vitamin D, essential for hormone production.

Chicken: Chicken provides lean protein necessary for energy and stamina. It also contains B vitamins that help maintain healthy energy levels.

Whole Grains

Oats: Oats improve blood flow and contain L-arginine, an amino acid that can enhance erectile function. They are also a great source of fiber, which supports overall health.

Quinoa: Quinoa is a complete protein, providing all essential amino acids. It also contains magnesium and potassium, which support cardiovascular health and blood flow.

Herbs and Spices

Garlic: Garlic contains allicin, which can improve blood flow and circulation. It also has anti-inflammatory properties that support overall health.

Ginseng: Ginseng is known for boosting libido and improving sexual performance. It also helps reduce stress and improve energy levels.

Fenugreek: Fenugreek may help increase libido and testosterone levels. It also contains fiber and antioxidants that support overall health.

Healthy Fats

Olive Oil: Olive oil improves circulation and heart health. It also contains healthy fats that support hormone production.

Nuts: Nuts provide essential fatty acids that support hormone production and overall health. They also offer protein and fiber for sustained energy.

Dark Chocolate

Dark chocolate contains flavonoids, which improve circulation and blood flow. It also increases serotonin and dopamine levels, which can enhance mood and sexual pleasure.

Shellfish

Oysters: Oysters are extremely high in zinc, which is essential for testosterone production and healthy sperm. They also provide protein and other essential nutrients.

Legumes

Chickpeas: Chickpeas are rich in zinc and other nutrients that support reproductive health. They also provide protein and fiber for sustained energy.

Lentils: Lentils are a great source of protein, iron, and folate, all of which support sexual health and overall well-being.

Moderation: The Role of Red Wine

Red Wine: Red wine, in moderation, contains antioxidants that can help improve circulation and heart health. However, it's important to consume it in moderation, as excessive alcohol intake can negatively affect sexual health.

By incorporating these foods into your diet, you can support your sexual health and enjoy a variety of delicious and nutritious meals. Let's get started on this journey to better health and vitality!

CHAPTER 1: ENERGIZING BREAKFASTS

Recipe 1: Banana Almond Smoothie

Quick and Nutritious Start to the Day

This Banana Almond Smoothie is a perfect way to kickstart your day with a boost of energy and essential nutrients. Packed with potassium, vitamin B6, healthy fats, and protein, this smoothie supports testosterone production and overall sexual health.

Ingredients

- 2 ripe bananas
- 250 ml almond milk
- 30 grams almonds
- 1 tablespoon honey
- 1 teaspoon vanilla extract
- 5 ice cubes

Instructions

1. **Prepare the Ingredients:** Peel the bananas and break them into chunks. Measure out the almond milk, almonds, honey, and vanilla extract.

2. **Blend:** In a blender, combine the banana chunks, almond milk, almonds, honey, vanilla extract, and ice

cubes.

3. **Blend Until Smooth:** Blend the ingredients on high speed until the mixture is smooth and creamy.

4. **Serve:** Pour the smoothie into a glass and enjoy immediately.

Nutrition per Serving (Serves 2)

- **Calories:** 250 kcal
- **Protein:** 5 grams
- **Fat:** 10 grams
- **Carbohydrates:** 35 grams
- **Fiber:** 4 grams
- **Sugar:** 20 grams
- **Potassium:** 500 mg
- **Vitamin B6:** 0.4 mg

This smoothie is not only delicious but also provides a substantial amount of potassium and vitamin B6, both of which are crucial for energy and sexual health. Enjoy this quick and easy recipe to start your day on a healthy note!

Recipe 2: Walnut and Berry Oatmeal

A Wholesome and Satisfying Breakfast

This Walnut and Berry Oatmeal is a nutritious and filling breakfast option that supports sexual health. The combination of oats, walnuts, and berries provides a rich source of fiber, omega-3 fatty acids, antioxidants, and essential vitamins.

Ingredients

- 100 grams rolled oats
- 500 ml water or milk (dairy or plant-based)

- 50 grams walnuts, chopped
- 100 grams mixed berries (blueberries, strawberries, raspberries)
- 1 tablespoon honey
- 1 teaspoon cinnamon (optional)

Instructions

1. **Cook the Oats:** In a medium saucepan, bring the water or milk to a boil. Add the rolled oats, reduce the heat, and simmer for about 5 minutes, stirring occasionally until the oats are tender and the mixture has thickened.

2. **Prepare the Toppings:** While the oats are cooking, chop the walnuts and wash the berries.

3. **Combine and Serve:** Once the oats are cooked, pour them into a bowl. Top with chopped walnuts, mixed berries, and a drizzle of honey. Sprinkle with cinnamon if desired.

4. **Enjoy:** Serve immediately while warm.

Nutrition per Serving (Serves 2)

- **Calories:** 350 kcal
- **Protein:** 8 grams
- **Fat:** 15 grams
- **Carbohydrates:** 45 grams
- **Fiber:** 7 grams
- **Sugar:** 15 grams
- **Omega-3 Fatty Acids:** 1.5 grams
- **Vitamin C:** 20 mg

This wholesome oatmeal provides a balanced mix of complex carbohydrates, healthy fats, and proteins, making it a perfect start to your day. The antioxidants from the berries and the omega-3 fatty acids from the walnuts support overall health and vitality. Enjoy this satisfying breakfast to fuel your morning!

Recipe 3: Spinach and Feta Omelette

Protein-Packed Breakfast with Essential Nutrients

This Spinach and Feta Omelette is a delicious and nutritious way to start your day. Rich in protein, vitamins, and minerals, this omelette supports muscle health, energy levels, and overall well-being.

Ingredients

- 4 large eggs
- 100 grams fresh spinach, washed and chopped
- 50 grams feta cheese, crumbled
- 1 small onion, finely chopped
- 1 clove garlic, minced
- 2 tablespoons olive oil
- Salt and pepper to taste

Instructions

1. **Prepare the Ingredients:** Crack the eggs into a bowl and whisk until well beaten. Chop the spinach, finely chop the onion, and mince the garlic.

2. **Sauté the Vegetables:** Heat 1 tablespoon of olive oil in a non-stick skillet over medium heat. Add the onion and garlic, and sauté until soft and translucent, about 3-4 minutes. Add the chopped spinach and cook until wilted, about 2 minutes.

3. **Cook the Omelette:** Remove the vegetables from the skillet and set aside. Add the remaining 1 tablespoon of olive oil to the skillet. Pour in the beaten eggs and cook

until the edges start to set, about 2 minutes.

4. **Add the Fillings:** Sprinkle the cooked spinach mixture and crumbled feta cheese evenly over one half of the omelette. Season with salt and pepper.

5. **Fold and Finish:** Carefully fold the omelette in half to cover the fillings. Cook for another 1-2 minutes until the eggs are fully set.

6. **Serve:** Slide the omelette onto a plate and serve immediately.

Nutrition per Serving (Serves 2)

- **Calories:** 300 kcal
- **Protein:** 18 grams
- **Fat:** 24 grams
- **Carbohydrates:** 5 grams
- **Fiber:** 2 grams
- **Sugar:** 2 grams
- **Vitamin A:** 3000 IU
- **Calcium:** 200 mg

This protein-packed omelette is not only delicious but also provides essential nutrients such as vitamin A, calcium, and iron. The combination of spinach and feta adds a flavorful and nutritious twist, making this an ideal breakfast to start your day with energy and vitality. Enjoy!

Recipe 4: Avocado and Walnut Smoothie

Creamy and Nutrient-Dense Smoothie to Fuel Your Morning

This Avocado and Walnut Smoothie is a creamy and delicious way to start your day. Packed with healthy fats, fiber, and essential vitamins, this smoothie supports heart health and provides sustained energy.

Ingredients

- 1 ripe avocado
- 250 ml almond milk
- 30 grams walnuts
- 1 tablespoon honey
- 1 small banana
- 1 teaspoon vanilla extract
- 5 ice cubes

Instructions

1. **Prepare the Ingredients:** Halve and pit the avocado, then scoop out the flesh. Peel and slice the banana.
2. **Blend:** In a blender, combine the avocado, almond milk, walnuts, honey, banana, vanilla extract, and ice cubes.
3. **Blend Until Smooth:** Blend the ingredients on high speed until the mixture is smooth and creamy.
4. **Serve:** Pour the smoothie into a glass and enjoy immediately.

Nutrition per Serving (Serves 2)

- **Calories:** 320 kcal
- **Protein:** 5 grams
- **Fat:** 23 grams
- **Carbohydrates:** 26 grams
- **Fiber:** 7 grams
- **Sugar:** 15 grams
- **Potassium:** 500 mg
- **Vitamin E:** 6 mg

This smoothie provides a rich source of healthy fats from the avocado and walnuts, along with the natural sweetness of banana and honey. It's perfect for a quick breakfast or a mid-morning snack to keep you energized and satisfied. Enjoy this nutrient-dense smoothie to fuel your day!

Recipe 5: Walnut and Banana Smoothie

Filling and Energy-Boosting Smoothie

This Walnut and Banana Smoothie is a perfect blend of protein, healthy fats, and natural sugars to provide a quick and energizing start to your day. It's ideal for a breakfast on the go or a nutritious snack.

Ingredients

- 2 ripe bananas
- 250 ml almond milk
- 30 grams walnuts
- 1 tablespoon honey
- 1 teaspoon cinnamon (optional)
- 5 ice cubes

Instructions

1. **Prepare the Ingredients:** Peel the bananas and break them into chunks. Measure out the almond milk, walnuts, honey, and cinnamon if using.

2. **Blend:** In a blender, combine the banana chunks, almond milk, walnuts, honey, cinnamon, and ice cubes.

3. **Blend Until Smooth:** Blend the ingredients on high speed until the mixture is smooth and creamy.

4. **Serve:** Pour the smoothie into a glass and enjoy immediately.

Nutrition per Serving (Serves 2)

- **Calories:** 280 kcal
- **Protein:** 5 grams
- **Fat:** 12 grams
- **Carbohydrates:** 42 grams
- **Fiber:** 4 grams
- **Sugar:** 25 grams
- **Potassium:** 600 mg
- **Magnesium:** 50 mg

This smoothie offers a balance of carbohydrates for energy, protein for muscle health, and healthy fats for sustained fullness. The combination of bananas and walnuts ensures a nutrient-dense and satisfying drink. Enjoy this filling smoothie to boost your energy levels!

CHAPTER 2: REFRESHING SALADS

Recipe 6: Watermelon Mint Salad

A Refreshing and Hydrating Salad

This Watermelon Mint Salad is a light, refreshing, and hydrating dish perfect for hot days. The combination of sweet watermelon and cool mint not only tastes great but also provides essential vitamins and antioxidants.

Ingredients

- 500 grams watermelon, cubed
- 20 grams fresh mint leaves, chopped
- 50 grams feta cheese, crumbled
- 1 tablespoon olive oil
- 1 tablespoon fresh lime juice
- Salt to taste

Instructions

1. **Prepare the Ingredients:** Cut the watermelon into bite-sized cubes. Chop the mint leaves and crumble the feta cheese.

2. **Combine:** In a large bowl, combine the watermelon cubes, chopped mint leaves, and crumbled feta cheese.

3. **Dress:** Drizzle the salad with olive oil and fresh lime juice. Add a pinch of salt to taste.

4. **Toss and Serve:** Gently toss the ingredients until well combined. Serve immediately.

Nutrition per Serving (Serves 4)

- **Calories:** 110 kcal
- **Protein:** 3 grams
- **Fat:** 6 grams
- **Carbohydrates:** 13 grams
- **Fiber:** 1 gram
- **Sugar:** 10 grams
- **Vitamin C:** 15 mg
- **Calcium:** 80 mg

This refreshing salad provides a great balance of hydration from the watermelon, healthy fats from the olive oil, and a touch of protein from the feta cheese. The mint adds a burst of freshness, making this a perfect light side dish or snack. Enjoy this hydrating salad to stay cool and nourished!

Recipe 7: Avocado and Pumpkin Seed Salad

Nutrient-Packed Salad with Healthy Fats

This Avocado and Pumpkin Seed Salad is a delicious and nutrient-dense dish that provides a wealth of healthy fats, vitamins, and minerals. It's a perfect meal for maintaining energy levels and supporting overall health.

Ingredients

- 1 large avocado
- 150 grams mixed greens (spinach, arugula, lettuce)
- 50 grams pumpkin seeds
- 100 grams cherry tomatoes, halved

- 1 small cucumber, sliced
- 2 tablespoons olive oil
- 1 tablespoon balsamic vinegar
- Salt and pepper to taste

Instructions

1. **Prepare the Ingredients:** Halve and pit the avocado, then slice it into thin pieces. Halve the cherry tomatoes and slice the cucumber.

2. **Assemble the Salad:** In a large salad bowl, combine the mixed greens, cherry tomatoes, cucumber, and avocado slices.

3. **Add the Seeds:** Sprinkle the pumpkin seeds over the top of the salad.

4. **Dress the Salad:** Drizzle the salad with olive oil and balsamic vinegar. Season with salt and pepper to taste.

5. **Toss and Serve:** Gently toss the salad to combine all ingredients. Serve immediately.

Nutrition per Serving (Serves 2)

- **Calories:** 320 kcal
- **Protein:** 6 grams
- **Fat:** 28 grams
- **Carbohydrates:** 14 grams
- **Fiber:** 7 grams
- **Sugar:** 5 grams
- **Vitamin E:** 5 mg
- **Magnesium:** 70 mg

This nutrient-packed salad is rich in healthy fats from the avocado and pumpkin seeds, which are essential for hormone production and overall health. The mixed greens and vegetables provide additional vitamins and minerals, making this a well-rounded and satisfying meal. Enjoy this delicious salad to boost your nutrient intake and stay energized!

Recipe 8: Spinach and Walnut Pesto Pasta

A Quick Pasta Salad with a Healthy Twist

This Spinach and Walnut Pesto Pasta is a delicious and healthy meal that combines the goodness of spinach and walnuts with the comfort of pasta. It's a perfect dish for a quick lunch or dinner, packed with essential nutrients and flavors.

Ingredients

- 200 grams whole wheat pasta
- 100 grams fresh spinach
- 50 grams walnuts
- 50 grams Parmesan cheese, grated
- 1 clove garlic
- 60 ml olive oil
- 1 tablespoon lemon juice
- Salt and pepper to taste
- Cherry tomatoes for garnish (optional)

Instructions

1. **Cook the Pasta:** Bring a large pot of salted water to a boil. Add the whole wheat pasta and cook according to package instructions until al dente. Drain and set aside.

2. **Prepare the Pesto:** In a food processor, combine the fresh spinach, walnuts, Parmesan cheese, garlic, olive oil, and lemon juice. Blend until smooth. Season with salt and pepper to taste.

3. **Combine Pasta and Pesto:** In a large bowl, toss the cooked pasta with the spinach and walnut pesto until well coated.

4. **Serve:** Garnish with cherry tomatoes if desired. Serve immediately.

Nutrition per Serving (Serves 2)

- **Calories:** 550 kcal
- **Protein:** 16 grams
- **Fat:** 34 grams
- **Carbohydrates:** 45 grams
- **Fiber:** 8 grams
- **Sugar:** 3 grams
- **Vitamin A:** 3000 IU
- **Calcium:** 250 mg

This quick and healthy pasta dish provides a great balance of complex carbohydrates, healthy fats, and protein. The spinach and walnut pesto adds a nutrient-dense twist, rich in vitamins, minerals, and antioxidants. Enjoy this flavorful pasta salad as a satisfying and nutritious meal!

Recipe 9: Salmon and Spinach Salad

Protein-Rich Salad with Essential Vitamins

This Salmon and Spinach Salad is a nutrient-dense meal that combines the rich flavors of salmon with the freshness of spinach. Packed with protein, omega-3 fatty acids, and essential vitamins, this salad supports overall health and vitality.

Ingredients

- 200 grams salmon fillet
- 150 grams fresh spinach

- 50 grams cherry tomatoes, halved
- 1 small red onion, thinly sliced
- 1 avocado, sliced
- 1 tablespoon olive oil
- 1 tablespoon lemon juice
- Salt and pepper to taste
- 1 teaspoon dried dill

Instructions

1. **Prepare the Salmon:** Preheat the oven to 200°C (400°F). Place the salmon fillet on a baking sheet lined with parchment paper. Drizzle with 1 teaspoon of olive oil, and season with salt, pepper, and dried dill. Bake for 12-15 minutes, or until the salmon is cooked through and flakes easily with a fork. Let it cool slightly and then break it into chunks.

2. **Prepare the Salad:** In a large salad bowl, combine the fresh spinach, cherry tomatoes, red onion, and avocado slices.

3. **Add the Salmon:** Add the cooked salmon chunks to the salad.

4. **Dress the Salad:** In a small bowl, whisk together the remaining olive oil and lemon juice. Drizzle over the salad and toss gently to combine.

5. **Serve:** Season with additional salt and pepper if needed. Serve immediately.

Nutrition per Serving (Serves 2)

- **Calories:** 400 kcal
- **Protein:** 28 grams
- **Fat:** 25 grams
- **Carbohydrates:** 10 grams

- **Fiber:** 5 grams
- **Sugar:** 3 grams
- **Omega-3 Fatty Acids:** 1.8 grams
- **Vitamin A:** 5000 IU
- **Vitamin C:** 20 mg

This protein-rich salad provides a substantial amount of omega-3 fatty acids from the salmon, as well as essential vitamins from the fresh vegetables. The combination of flavors and textures makes this a delicious and satisfying meal. Enjoy this wholesome salad for a boost of energy and nutrition!

Recipe 10: Avocado and Spinach Salad

Refreshing and Light Salad for Any Meal

This Avocado and Spinach Salad is a light and refreshing dish perfect for any meal. Packed with healthy fats, vitamins, and minerals, this salad supports overall health and vitality.

Ingredients

- 150 grams fresh spinach
- 1 large avocado, sliced
- 50 grams cherry tomatoes, halved
- 1 small red onion, thinly sliced
- 1 tablespoon olive oil
- 1 tablespoon lemon juice
- Salt and pepper to taste

Instructions

1. **Prepare the Ingredients:** Wash and dry the spinach. Slice the avocado, halve the cherry tomatoes, and thinly slice the red onion.

2. **Assemble the Salad:** In a large salad bowl, combine the fresh spinach, avocado slices, cherry tomatoes, and red onion.

3. **Dress the Salad:** In a small bowl, whisk together the olive oil and lemon juice. Drizzle over the salad and toss gently to combine.

4. **Serve:** Season with salt and pepper to taste. Serve immediately.

Nutrition per Serving (Serves 2)

- **Calories:** 220 kcal
- **Protein:** 3 grams
- **Fat:** 20 grams
- **Carbohydrates:** 10 grams
- **Fiber:** 7 grams
- **Sugar:** 2 grams
- **Vitamin A:** 4000 IU
- **Vitamin C:** 20 mg
- **Potassium:** 600 mg

This refreshing and light salad provides a great balance of healthy fats from the avocado and essential vitamins from the spinach and tomatoes. It's perfect as a side dish or a light meal, offering a burst of flavor and nutrition. Enjoy this simple and delicious salad for a quick and healthy option!

CHAPTER 3: NUTRITIOUS MAIN DISHES

Recipe 11: Salmon and Avocado Sushi Rolls

Easy-to-Make Sushi Rolls Packed with Omega-3s

These Salmon and Avocado Sushi Rolls are a delicious and nutritious way to enjoy sushi at home. Packed with omega-3 fatty acids from the salmon and healthy fats from the avocado, these sushi rolls are both satisfying and good for you.

Ingredients

- 200 grams sushi-grade salmon, thinly sliced
- 1 large avocado, sliced
- 250 grams sushi rice
- 3 tablespoons rice vinegar
- 1 tablespoon sugar
- 1 teaspoon salt
- 4 nori sheets (seaweed)
- Soy sauce for dipping
- Pickled ginger and wasabi for serving (optional)

Instructions

1. **Prepare the Sushi Rice:** Rinse the sushi rice under cold

water until the water runs clear. Cook the rice according to the package instructions. In a small bowl, mix the rice vinegar, sugar, and salt until dissolved. Once the rice is cooked, gently fold in the vinegar mixture. Allow the rice to cool to room temperature.

2. **Prepare the Ingredients:** Thinly slice the sushi-grade salmon and the avocado.

3. **Assemble the Sushi Rolls:** Place a nori sheet on a bamboo sushi mat, shiny side down. Spread a thin layer of sushi rice over the nori, leaving a 2 cm border at the top edge. Arrange a few slices of salmon and avocado horizontally across the center of the rice.

4. **Roll the Sushi:** Using the bamboo mat, roll the nori and rice over the fillings, applying gentle pressure to form a tight roll. Seal the roll by moistening the top border of the nori with water. Repeat with the remaining ingredients.

5. **Slice and Serve:** Using a sharp knife, slice each roll into 6-8 pieces. Serve with soy sauce, pickled ginger, and wasabi if desired.

Nutrition per Serving (Serves 4)

- **Calories:** 350 kcal

- **Protein:** 15 grams

- **Fat:** 15 grams

- **Carbohydrates:** 40 grams

- **Fiber:** 5 grams

- **Sugar:** 3 grams

- **Omega-3 Fatty Acids:** 1.5 grams

- **Vitamin A:** 200 IU

- **Vitamin C:** 6 mg

These easy-to-make sushi rolls are not only delicious but also provide a good dose of omega-3 fatty acids, which are essential for heart health. The combination of salmon and avocado offers a creamy and flavorful experience. Enjoy these sushi rolls as a healthy and tasty meal or snack!

Recipe 12: Garlic Shrimp Stir-Fry

Quick and Flavorful Stir-Fry

This Garlic Shrimp Stir-Fry is a quick and delicious meal that's full of flavor and nutrients. The shrimp provides a good source of protein and omega-3 fatty acids, while the garlic adds a boost of antioxidants.

Ingredients

- 300 grams shrimp, peeled and deveined
- 1 red bell pepper, sliced
- 1 yellow bell pepper, sliced
- 1 small broccoli, cut into florets
- 1 carrot, sliced
- 4 cloves garlic, minced
- 2 tablespoons olive oil
- 2 tablespoons soy sauce
- 1 tablespoon honey
- 1 teaspoon grated ginger
- 1 tablespoon sesame seeds (optional)
- 2 green onions, sliced (optional)
- Cooked rice or noodles, for serving

Instructions

1. **Prepare the Sauce:** In a small bowl, mix the soy sauce,

honey, and grated ginger. Set aside.

2. **Cook the Shrimp:** Heat 1 tablespoon of olive oil in a large skillet or wok over medium-high heat. Add the shrimp and cook until pink and opaque, about 2-3 minutes per side. Remove the shrimp from the skillet and set aside.

3. **Stir-Fry the Vegetables:** In the same skillet, add the remaining olive oil. Add the minced garlic and sauté for about 30 seconds until fragrant. Add the sliced bell peppers, broccoli florets, and carrot. Stir-fry for about 5-7 minutes until the vegetables are tender-crisp.

4. **Combine and Serve:** Return the cooked shrimp to the skillet. Pour the sauce over the shrimp and vegetables and stir to coat evenly. Cook for an additional 2 minutes until everything is heated through. Sprinkle with sesame seeds and green onions if desired. Serve immediately over cooked rice or noodles.

Nutrition per Serving (Serves 4)

- **Calories:** 250 kcal
- **Protein:** 20 grams
- **Fat:** 10 grams
- **Carbohydrates:** 20 grams
- **Fiber:** 4 grams
- **Sugar:** 7 grams
- **Vitamin C:** 60 mg
- **Iron:** 3 mg

This quick and flavorful stir-fry is perfect for a busy weeknight. The combination of shrimp and vegetables provides a balanced meal that is both nutritious and delicious. Enjoy this healthy stir-fry with a side of rice or noodles for a complete meal!

Recipe 13: Ginger and Garlic Chicken

Zesty and Aromatic Chicken Dish

This Ginger and Garlic Chicken is a zesty and aromatic dish that's packed with flavor. The combination of ginger and garlic not only adds a delicious taste but also provides numerous health benefits, including anti-inflammatory and immune-boosting properties.

Ingredients

- 400 grams chicken breast, cut into bite-sized pieces
- 4 cloves garlic, minced
- 2 tablespoons fresh ginger, grated
- 2 tablespoons soy sauce
- 1 tablespoon honey
- 1 tablespoon olive oil
- 1 tablespoon sesame oil
- 1 red bell pepper, sliced
- 1 green bell pepper, sliced
- 1 small onion, sliced
- 1 tablespoon sesame seeds (optional)
- Cooked rice or noodles, for serving

Instructions

1. **Marinate the Chicken:** In a bowl, combine the minced garlic, grated ginger, soy sauce, and honey. Add the chicken pieces and toss to coat. Let it marinate for at least 15 minutes.

2. **Cook the Chicken:** Heat the olive oil and sesame oil in a large skillet or wok over medium-high heat. Add the marinated chicken and cook until browned and cooked

through, about 6-8 minutes. Remove the chicken from the skillet and set aside.

3. **Stir-Fry the Vegetables:** In the same skillet, add the sliced bell peppers and onion. Stir-fry for about 4-5 minutes until the vegetables are tender-crisp.

4. **Combine and Serve:** Return the cooked chicken to the skillet. Toss everything together until well combined and heated through. Sprinkle with sesame seeds if desired. Serve immediately over cooked rice or noodles.

Nutrition per Serving (Serves 4)

- **Calories:** 300 kcal
- **Protein:** 25 grams
- **Fat:** 12 grams
- **Carbohydrates:** 20 grams
- **Fiber:** 3 grams
- **Sugar:** 8 grams
- **Vitamin C:** 70 mg
- **Iron:** 2 mg

This zesty and aromatic chicken dish is perfect for a flavorful and healthy meal. The ginger and garlic not only add a punch of flavor but also offer numerous health benefits. Enjoy this dish over a bed of rice or noodles for a complete and satisfying meal!

Recipe 14: Walnut-Crusted Salmon

Crispy and Flavorful Salmon

This Walnut-Crusted Salmon is a delicious and nutritious dish that's crispy on the outside and tender on the inside. The walnuts add a rich, nutty flavor and a satisfying crunch, making this a perfect meal for any occasion.

Ingredients

- 4 salmon fillets (about 150 grams each)
- 100 grams walnuts, finely chopped
- 2 tablespoons Dijon mustard
- 1 tablespoon honey
- 1 tablespoon olive oil
- 1 teaspoon fresh thyme, chopped (optional)
- Salt and pepper to taste
- Lemon wedges, for serving

Instructions

1. **Preheat the Oven:** Preheat your oven to 200°C (400°F). Line a baking sheet with parchment paper.
2. **Prepare the Salmon:** Place the salmon fillets on the prepared baking sheet. Season with salt and pepper.
3. **Make the Walnut Crust:** In a small bowl, combine the finely chopped walnuts, Dijon mustard, honey, olive oil, and fresh thyme (if using). Mix well to form a paste.
4. **Crust the Salmon:** Spread the walnut mixture evenly over the top of each salmon fillet, pressing down gently to adhere.
5. **Bake the Salmon:** Bake in the preheated oven for 12-15 minutes, or until the salmon is cooked through and the walnut crust is golden and crispy.
6. **Serve:** Serve the walnut-crusted salmon with lemon wedges on the side.

Nutrition per Serving (Serves 4)

- **Calories:** 420 kcal
- **Protein:** 28 grams
- **Fat:** 30 grams
- **Carbohydrates:** 8 grams

- **Fiber:** 2 grams
- **Sugar:** 5 grams
- **Omega-3 Fatty Acids:** 1.8 grams
- **Vitamin D:** 400 IU
- **Selenium:** 35 mcg

This walnut-crusted salmon is not only delicious but also provides a great source of omega-3 fatty acids, which are essential for heart health. The combination of flavors and textures makes this dish both satisfying and nutritious. Enjoy this crispy and flavorful salmon for a healthy and tasty meal!

Recipe 15: Salmon and Quinoa Bowl

Balanced Bowl with Protein and Healthy Grains

This Salmon and Quinoa Bowl is a balanced and nutritious meal that combines protein-rich salmon with fiber-packed quinoa and fresh vegetables. It's a wholesome dish that provides essential nutrients to support your overall health and well-being.

Ingredients

- 300 grams salmon fillets
- 150 grams quinoa
- 1 tablespoon olive oil
- 1 garlic clove, minced
- 1 small zucchini, diced
- 1 bell pepper, diced
- 1 cup cherry tomatoes, halved
- 2 tablespoons lemon juice
- Salt and pepper to taste
- Fresh parsley or cilantro for garnish (optional)

Instructions

1. **Cook the Quinoa:** Rinse the quinoa under cold water. In a medium saucepan, bring 2 cups of water to a boil. Add the quinoa, reduce heat to low, cover, and simmer for 15 minutes or until the quinoa is cooked and water is absorbed. Fluff with a fork and set aside.

2. **Prepare the Salmon:** Season the salmon fillets with salt and pepper. In a large skillet, heat olive oil over medium-high heat. Add the salmon fillets, skin side down, and cook for about 4-5 minutes per side, or until cooked through and easily flakes with a fork. Remove from heat and let it rest for a few minutes. Remove the skin and break into large chunks.

3. **Sauté the Vegetables:** In the same skillet used for the salmon, add minced garlic, diced zucchini, and bell pepper. Sauté for about 3-4 minutes until vegetables are tender-crisp. Add cherry tomatoes and cook for an additional 1-2 minutes.

4. **Assemble the Bowl:** Divide cooked quinoa among serving bowls. Top with sautéed vegetables and salmon chunks. Drizzle with lemon juice. Season with additional salt and pepper if needed. Garnish with fresh parsley or cilantro if desired.

5. **Serve:** Serve immediately and enjoy this balanced and nutritious salmon and quinoa bowl!

Nutrition per Serving (Serves 2)

- **Calories:** 450 kcal

- **Protein:** 35 grams

- **Fat:** 20 grams

- **Carbohydrates:** 30 grams

- **Fiber:** 5 grams

- **Sugar:** 5 grams
- **Omega-3 Fatty Acids:** 1.5 grams
- **Vitamin C:** 60 mg
- **Iron:** 3 mg

This salmon and quinoa bowl provides a perfect balance of protein, healthy fats, and complex carbohydrates. It's packed with vitamins, minerals, and antioxidants from the vegetables, making it a nutritious and satisfying meal option. Enjoy this wholesome bowl for lunch or dinner to fuel your body with essential nutrients!

CHAPTER 4:
SIMPLE SIDES

Recipe 16: Garlic and Lemon Roasted Broccoli

Easy and Delicious Roasted Broccoli

This Garlic and Lemon Roasted Broccoli is a simple yet flavorful side dish that pairs well with any main course. Roasting broccoli enhances its natural sweetness and the addition of garlic and lemon adds a zesty twist.

Ingredients

- 500 grams broccoli florets
- 3 cloves garlic, minced
- Zest of 1 lemon
- 2 tablespoons olive oil
- Salt and pepper to taste
- Lemon wedges for serving (optional)

Instructions

1. **Preheat the Oven:** Preheat your oven to 200°C (400°F). Line a baking sheet with parchment paper.

2. **Prepare the Broccoli:** Wash and dry the broccoli florets. Trim any tough stems and cut into bite-sized pieces.

3. **Toss with Seasonings:** In a large bowl, toss the broccoli florets with minced garlic, lemon zest, olive oil, salt, and pepper until evenly coated.

4. **Roast the Broccoli:** Spread the seasoned broccoli florets in a single layer on the prepared baking sheet.

5. **Roast in the Oven:** Roast in the preheated oven for 20-25 minutes, tossing halfway through, until the broccoli is tender and lightly browned on the edges.

6. **Serve:** Transfer the roasted broccoli to a serving dish. Squeeze fresh lemon juice over the top if desired. Serve hot as a delicious and nutritious side dish.

Nutrition per Serving (Serves 4)

- **Calories:** 120 kcal
- **Protein:** 5 grams
- **Fat:** 7 grams
- **Carbohydrates:** 12 grams
- **Fiber:** 5 grams
- **Sugar:** 3 grams
- **Vitamin C:** 120 mg
- **Calcium:** 70 mg

This easy and delicious roasted broccoli dish is packed with vitamins, minerals, and fiber. The garlic and lemon add a delightful flavor that complements the natural sweetness of the roasted broccoli. Enjoy this nutritious side dish with your favorite main course!

Recipe 17: Garlic and Almond Green Beans

Crunchy and Flavorful Green Beans

These Garlic and Almond Green Beans are a simple yet tasty side dish that pairs well with a variety of main courses. The combination of garlic and almonds adds a delicious crunch and nutty flavor to the tender green beans.

Ingredients

- 400 grams green beans, trimmed
- 2 cloves garlic, minced
- 50 grams almonds, sliced or slivered
- 2 tablespoons olive oil
- Salt and pepper to taste
- Lemon wedges for serving (optional)

Instructions

1. **Blanch the Green Beans:** Bring a large pot of salted water to a boil. Add the green beans and blanch for 2-3 minutes, until bright green and tender-crisp. Drain and immediately plunge the green beans into a bowl of ice water to stop the cooking process. Drain again and set aside.

2. **Toast the Almonds:** In a dry skillet over medium heat, toast the almonds until lightly golden and fragrant, about 2-3 minutes. Remove from the skillet and set aside.

3. **Sauté the Garlic:** In the same skillet, heat the olive oil over medium heat. Add the minced garlic and sauté for about 30 seconds until fragrant.

4. **Cook the Green Beans:** Add the blanched green beans to the skillet with the garlic. Toss to coat evenly with the garlic-infused oil. Cook for another 2-3 minutes, stirring occasionally, until the green beans are heated through and tender.

5. **Combine with Almonds:** Add the toasted almonds to the skillet with the green beans. Toss to combine and cook for another minute to warm the almonds.

6. **Serve:** Season with salt and pepper to taste. Serve hot, garnished with lemon wedges if desired.

Nutrition per Serving (Serves 4)

- **Calories:** 150 kcal
- **Protein:** 5 grams
- **Fat:** 10 grams
- **Carbohydrates:** 12 grams
- **Fiber:** 5 grams
- **Sugar:** 3 grams
- **Vitamin C:** 20 mg
- **Calcium:** 80 mg

These crunchy and flavorful garlic and almond green beans are a perfect addition to any meal. They are packed with nutrients and offer a delicious way to enjoy green beans. Serve them alongside your favorite main dish for a healthy and satisfying meal!

Recipe 18: Garlic and Olive Oil Spaghetti

Simple and Satisfying Pasta Side

This Garlic and Olive Oil Spaghetti, also known as Aglio e Olio, is a classic Italian dish that's quick to make and bursting with flavor. It's perfect as a simple and satisfying pasta side or even as a light main course.

Ingredients

- 300 grams spaghetti
- 4 cloves garlic, thinly sliced
- 1/3 cup olive oil
- 1/2 teaspoon red pepper flakes (adjust to taste)
- Salt and pepper to taste
- Fresh parsley, chopped, for garnish (optional)

- Grated Parmesan cheese, for serving (optional)

Instructions

1. **Cook the Spaghetti:** Cook the spaghetti in a large pot of salted boiling water according to the package instructions until al dente. Reserve about 1/2 cup of pasta water before draining.

2. **Prepare the Garlic Sauce:** While the spaghetti is cooking, heat the olive oil in a large skillet over medium heat. Add the thinly sliced garlic and red pepper flakes. Sauté for about 2-3 minutes, stirring occasionally, until the garlic is golden brown and fragrant. Be careful not to burn the garlic.

3. **Combine the Pasta:** Once the spaghetti is cooked, add it directly to the skillet with the garlic oil. Toss to coat the spaghetti evenly with the garlic sauce. If needed, add a splash of reserved pasta water to loosen the sauce.

4. **Season and Serve:** Season with salt and pepper to taste. Garnish with chopped fresh parsley if desired. Serve hot, with grated Parmesan cheese on the side if desired.

Nutrition per Serving (Serves 4)

- **Calories:** 400 kcal
- **Protein:** 8 grams
- **Fat:** 20 grams
- **Carbohydrates:** 50 grams
- **Fiber:** 3 grams
- **Sugar:** 2 grams
- **Vitamin C:** 2 mg
- **Calcium:** 20 mg

This simple and satisfying garlic and olive oil spaghetti is a staple in Italian cuisine. It's quick to prepare yet full of flavor, making it a perfect dish for busy weeknights or any occasion. Enjoy this classic pasta side with a fresh salad or as a complement to your favorite main dish!

Recipe 19: Garlic and Olive Oil Spaghetti

Simple and Satisfying Pasta Side

This Garlic and Olive Oil Spaghetti, also known as Aglio e Olio, is a classic Italian dish that's quick to make and bursting with flavor. It's perfect as a simple and satisfying pasta side or even as a light main course.

Ingredients

- 300 grams spaghetti
- 4 cloves garlic, thinly sliced
- 1/3 cup olive oil
- 1/2 teaspoon red pepper flakes (adjust to taste)
- Salt and pepper to taste
- Fresh parsley, chopped, for garnish (optional)
- Grated Parmesan cheese, for serving (optional)

Instructions

1. **Cook the Spaghetti:** Cook the spaghetti in a large pot of salted boiling water according to the package instructions until al dente. Reserve about 1/2 cup of pasta water before draining.

2. **Prepare the Garlic Sauce:** While the spaghetti is cooking, heat the olive oil in a large skillet over medium heat. Add the thinly sliced garlic and red pepper flakes. Sauté for about 2-3 minutes, stirring occasionally, until the garlic is golden brown and fragrant. Be careful not to burn the garlic.

3. **Combine the Pasta:** Once the spaghetti is cooked, add it

directly to the skillet with the garlic oil. Toss to coat the spaghetti evenly with the garlic sauce. If needed, add a splash of reserved pasta water to loosen the sauce.

4. **Season and Serve:** Season with salt and pepper to taste. Garnish with chopped fresh parsley if desired. Serve hot, with grated Parmesan cheese on the side if desired.

Nutrition per Serving (Serves 4)

- **Calories:** 400 kcal
- **Protein:** 8 grams
- **Fat:** 20 grams
- **Carbohydrates:** 50 grams
- **Fiber:** 3 grams
- **Sugar:** 2 grams
- **Vitamin C:** 2 mg
- **Calcium:** 20 mg

This simple and satisfying garlic and olive oil spaghetti is a staple in Italian cuisine. It's quick to prepare yet full of flavor, making it a perfect dish for busy weeknights or any occasion. Enjoy this classic pasta side with a fresh salad or as a complement to your favorite main dish!

Recipe 20: Garlic and Lemon Shrimp Skewers

Quick and Tasty Shrimp Skewers

These Garlic and Lemon Shrimp Skewers are a flavorful and easy-to-make dish that's perfect for grilling or cooking indoors. The combination of garlic, lemon, and shrimp creates a zesty and delicious meal that's sure to please.

Ingredients

- 400 grams large shrimp, peeled and deveined

- Zest and juice of 1 lemon
- 3 cloves garlic, minced
- 2 tablespoons olive oil
- 1 tablespoon chopped fresh parsley
- Salt and pepper to taste
- Lemon wedges for serving

Instructions

1. **Marinate the Shrimp:** In a bowl, combine the olive oil, minced garlic, lemon zest, lemon juice, chopped parsley, salt, and pepper. Add the shrimp and toss to coat evenly. Marinate for at least 15 minutes, or up to 30 minutes in the refrigerator.

2. **Prepare the Skewers:** If using wooden skewers, soak them in water for 15-20 minutes to prevent burning. Thread the marinated shrimp onto skewers, leaving a little space between each shrimp.

3. **Grill or Cook the Skewers:** Preheat the grill or a grill pan over medium-high heat. Grill the shrimp skewers for about 2-3 minutes per side, or until shrimp are opaque and cooked through. Alternatively, you can cook them in a skillet over medium-high heat for the same amount of time.

4. **Serve:** Remove the shrimp skewers from the grill or skillet. Serve hot, garnished with lemon wedges for squeezing over the shrimp.

Nutrition per Serving (Serves 4)

- **Calories:** 200 kcal
- **Protein:** 25 grams
- **Fat:** 9 grams
- **Carbohydrates:** 2 grams

- **Fiber:** 0 grams
- **Sugar:** 0 grams
- **Vitamin C:** 15 mg
- **Iron:** 2 mg

These quick and tasty garlic and lemon shrimp skewers are perfect for a light and flavorful meal. They're easy to prepare and cook quickly, making them ideal for busy weeknights or summer grilling sessions. Enjoy these delicious shrimp skewers with a side of salad or grilled vegetables!

CHAPTER 5: HEALTHY SNACKS AND TREATS

Recipe 21: Pumpkin Seed and Dark Chocolate Bark

Sweet and Healthy Snack

This Pumpkin Seed and Dark Chocolate Bark combines the richness of dark chocolate with the crunchiness of pumpkin seeds, creating a delicious and nutritious snack that's easy to make and enjoy.

Ingredients

- 200 grams dark chocolate (70% cocoa or higher), chopped
- 50 grams pumpkin seeds
- 1/4 teaspoon sea salt flakes (optional)

Instructions

1. **Melt the Chocolate:** Line a baking sheet with parchment paper. Place the chopped dark chocolate in a microwave-safe bowl or double boiler. Microwave in 30-second intervals, stirring in between, until the chocolate is melted and smooth.

2. **Prepare the Bark:** Pour the melted chocolate onto the prepared baking sheet. Use a spatula to spread the chocolate evenly into a thin layer, about 1/4-inch thick.

3. **Add Pumpkin Seeds:** Sprinkle the pumpkin seeds evenly over the melted chocolate. Press them gently into the

chocolate.

4. **Set the Bark:** If using sea salt flakes, sprinkle them lightly over the chocolate bark.

5. **Chill and Break:** Transfer the baking sheet to the refrigerator and chill for about 30 minutes, or until the chocolate is firm. Once set, break the bark into pieces of desired sizes.

6. **Serve:** Serve the pumpkin seed and dark chocolate bark as a sweet and healthy snack. Store any leftovers in an airtight container at room temperature.

Nutrition per Serving (Makes about 10 servings)

- **Calories:** 150 kcal
- **Protein:** 3 grams
- **Fat:** 10 grams
- **Carbohydrates:** 15 grams
- **Fiber:** 3 grams
- **Sugar:** 8 grams
- **Iron:** 3 mg

This pumpkin seed and dark chocolate bark is a satisfying treat that combines the antioxidant-rich benefits of dark chocolate with the nutritious crunch of pumpkin seeds. Enjoy it as a guilt-free snack or dessert option!

Recipe 22: Avocado Chocolate Pudding

Creamy and Healthy Dessert

This Avocado Chocolate Pudding is a rich and creamy dessert that's surprisingly healthy, thanks to the natural creaminess of avocado and the indulgence of dark chocolate. It's a guilt-free treat that's easy to make and sure to satisfy your chocolate cravings.

Ingredients

- 2 ripe avocados
- 100 grams dark chocolate (70% cocoa or higher), melted
- 3 tablespoons cocoa powder
- 4 tablespoons maple syrup or honey (adjust to taste)
- 1 teaspoon vanilla extract
- Pinch of sea salt
- Fresh berries or chopped nuts for garnish (optional)

Instructions

1. **Prepare the Avocados:** Cut the avocados in half, remove the pits, and scoop the flesh into a food processor or blender.

2. **Blend Ingredients:** Add the melted dark chocolate, cocoa powder, maple syrup or honey, vanilla extract, and a pinch of sea salt to the avocados. Blend until smooth and creamy, scraping down the sides as needed to ensure everything is well combined.

3. **Chill (optional):** For a thicker pudding, chill in the refrigerator for 30 minutes to 1 hour before serving.

4. **Serve:** Divide the avocado chocolate pudding into serving bowls or glasses. Garnish with fresh berries or chopped nuts if desired.

5. **Enjoy:** Serve chilled or at room temperature as a creamy and healthy dessert option.

Nutrition per Serving (Serves 4)

- **Calories:** 250 kcal
- **Protein:** 4 grams
- **Fat:** 18 grams
- **Carbohydrates:** 25 grams

- **Fiber:** 8 grams
- **Sugar:** 14 grams
- **Vitamin C:** 10 mg
- **Calcium:** 40 mg

This avocado chocolate pudding is not only delicious but also packed with healthy fats, fiber, and antioxidants. It's a perfect dessert for those looking to enjoy something sweet while maintaining a nutritious diet. Indulge in this creamy treat guilt-free!

Recipe 23: Dark Chocolate Dipped Strawberries

Sweet and Antioxidant-Rich Treat

These Dark Chocolate Dipped Strawberries are a simple yet elegant dessert that combines the sweetness of ripe strawberries with the richness of dark chocolate. They're perfect for special occasions or as a healthier indulgence.

Ingredients

- 200 grams dark chocolate (70% cocoa or higher), chopped
- 250 grams fresh strawberries, washed and dried

Instructions

1. **Prepare the Chocolate:** Line a baking sheet with parchment paper. Place the chopped dark chocolate in a microwave-safe bowl or double boiler. Microwave in 30-second intervals, stirring in between, until the chocolate is melted and smooth.

2. **Dip the Strawberries:** Hold each strawberry by the stem and dip it into the melted chocolate, swirling to coat about two-thirds of the strawberry. Allow any excess chocolate to drip back into the bowl.

3. **Set on Baking Sheet:** Place the dipped strawberries on the prepared baking sheet. Repeat with the remaining strawberries and chocolate.

4. **Chill (optional):** Place the baking sheet in the refrigerator for about 15-20 minutes, or until the chocolate is set.

5. **Serve:** Arrange the dark chocolate dipped strawberries on a serving platter. Serve immediately as a sweet and antioxidant-rich treat.

Nutrition per Serving (Serves 4, approximately 5 strawberries per serving)

- **Calories:** 150 kcal
- **Protein:** 2 grams
- **Fat:** 10 grams
- **Carbohydrates:** 15 grams
- **Fiber:** 4 grams
- **Sugar:** 10 grams
- **Vitamin C:** 60 mg
- **Iron:** 2 mg

These dark chocolate dipped strawberries are not only delicious but also provide a dose of antioxidants from both the dark chocolate and fresh strawberries. Enjoy them as a delightful dessert or a special treat for any occasion!

Recipe 24: Dark Chocolate and Pumpkin Seed Energy Bites

Nutritious and Energizing Snack

These Dark Chocolate and Pumpkin Seed Energy Bites are packed with wholesome ingredients to provide a boost of energy and satisfy your snack cravings. They're easy to make, portable, and perfect for a quick bite on the go.

Ingredients

- 100 grams rolled oats
- 50 grams pumpkin seeds
- 50 grams dark chocolate (70% cocoa or higher), chopped
- 50 grams almond butter or any nut butter of choice
- 3 tablespoons honey or maple syrup
- 1/2 teaspoon vanilla extract
- Pinch of sea salt

Instructions

1. **Combine Ingredients:** In a large bowl, combine rolled oats, pumpkin seeds, chopped dark chocolate, almond butter, honey or maple syrup, vanilla extract, and a pinch of sea salt. Mix well until all ingredients are evenly incorporated.

2. **Chill the Mixture:** Place the mixture in the refrigerator for 15-30 minutes to firm up slightly. This will make it easier to form into balls.

3. **Form Energy Bites:** Remove the mixture from the refrigerator. Using clean hands, scoop about a tablespoon of the mixture and roll it between your palms to form a ball. Repeat with the remaining mixture to make approximately 12-15 energy bites.

4. **Store:** Store the energy bites in an airtight container in the refrigerator for up to 1 week, or freeze for longer storage.

5. **Serve:** Enjoy these nutritious and energizing dark chocolate and pumpkin seed energy bites as a snack or a quick pick-me-up during the day.

Nutrition per Serving (Makes about 15 energy bites)

- **Calories:** 100 kcal
- **Protein:** 3 grams
- **Fat:** 6 grams
- **Carbohydrates:** 10 grams
- **Fiber:** 2 grams
- **Sugar:** 5 grams
- **Iron:** 1 mg

These dark chocolate and pumpkin seed energy bites are not only delicious but also packed with nutrients from oats, pumpkin seeds, and dark chocolate. They provide a balanced source of energy to keep you fueled throughout the day. Enjoy these wholesome snacks whenever you need a boost!

Recipe 25: Dark Chocolate Walnut Clusters

Simple and Satisfying Treat

These Dark Chocolate Walnut Clusters are a delightful combination of crunchy walnuts and rich dark chocolate, perfect for satisfying your sweet tooth or as a homemade gift.

Ingredients

- 150 grams dark chocolate (70% cocoa or higher), chopped
- 100 grams walnuts, roughly chopped

Instructions

1. **Melt the Chocolate:** Line a baking sheet with parchment paper. Place the chopped dark chocolate in a microwave-safe bowl or double boiler. Microwave in 30-second intervals, stirring in between, until the chocolate is melted and smooth.
2. **Mix Ingredients:** Add the roughly chopped walnuts to

the melted chocolate. Stir until the walnuts are evenly coated with chocolate.

3. **Form Clusters:** Using a spoon or your hands, scoop about a tablespoon of the chocolate-walnut mixture and drop it onto the prepared baking sheet, forming clusters. Leave space between each cluster.

4. **Chill and Set:** Place the baking sheet in the refrigerator for about 15-20 minutes, or until the chocolate is set.

5. **Serve:** Once set, peel the clusters off the parchment paper and transfer them to a serving plate or store in an airtight container.

Nutrition per Serving (Makes about 10 clusters)

- **Calories:** 150 kcal
- **Protein:** 3 grams
- **Fat:** 10 grams
- **Carbohydrates:** 12 grams
- **Fiber:** 3 grams
- **Sugar:** 8 grams
- **Iron:** 2 mg

These dark chocolate walnut clusters are a simple and satisfying treat that combines the crunch of walnuts with the richness of dark chocolate. Enjoy them as a delicious snack or serve them at parties for a homemade touch that everyone will love!

CHAPTER 6: LIGHT MEALS AND WRAPS

Recipe 26: Avocado and Spinach Toast

Quick and Easy Toast for Any Time of Day

This Avocado and Spinach Toast is a nutritious and satisfying meal or snack that can be enjoyed for breakfast, lunch, or a light dinner. Packed with healthy fats, vitamins, and minerals, it's simple to make and delicious to eat.

Ingredients

- 2 slices whole grain bread, toasted
- 1 ripe avocado
- 1 cup fresh spinach leaves
- 1 tablespoon lemon juice
- Salt and pepper to taste
- Red pepper flakes (optional)
- Toasted sesame seeds for garnish (optional)

Instructions

1. **Prepare Avocado Spread:** In a bowl, mash the ripe avocado with lemon juice until smooth. Season with salt, pepper, and red pepper flakes if using.

2. **Cook Spinach (optional):** If desired, quickly sauté the fresh spinach leaves in a pan with a little olive oil until wilted, about 1-2 minutes.

3. **Assemble the Toast:** Spread the mashed avocado evenly onto the toasted whole grain bread slices.

4. **Top with Spinach:** Arrange the sautéed spinach leaves on top of the avocado spread.

5. **Garnish and Serve:** Sprinkle with toasted sesame seeds for added crunch and flavor, if desired. Serve immediately.

Nutrition per Serving (2 slices of toast)

- **Calories:** 300 kcal
- **Protein:** 8 grams
- **Fat:** 15 grams
- **Carbohydrates:** 35 grams
- **Fiber:** 12 grams
- **Sugar:** 4 grams
- **Vitamin A:** 600 IU
- **Vitamin C:** 20 mg
- **Calcium:** 80 mg

This avocado and spinach toast is not only quick and easy to make but also provides a good balance of protein, healthy fats, and fiber. Enjoy it as a nutritious meal or snack any time of day!

Recipe 27: Fenugreek and Chickpea Salad

Light and Nutritious Salad

This Fenugreek and Chickpea Salad combines the unique flavors of fenugreek with the protein-packed goodness of chickpeas, creating a light and nutritious dish that's perfect as a side or a light meal.

Ingredients

- 200 grams cooked chickpeas (canned or boiled)
- 1 cup fresh fenugreek leaves, chopped (methi leaves)
- 1 small cucumber, diced
- 1 tomato, diced
- 1/4 cup red onion, finely chopped
- 2 tablespoons fresh lemon juice
- 2 tablespoons olive oil
- Salt and pepper to taste
- Fresh cilantro or parsley, chopped, for garnish (optional)

Instructions

1. **Prepare Chickpeas:** Rinse and drain the cooked chickpeas if using canned. If using dried chickpeas, cook according to package instructions until tender.

2. **Mix Ingredients:** In a large bowl, combine the chickpeas, chopped fenugreek leaves, diced cucumber, diced tomato, and finely chopped red onion.

3. **Dress the Salad:** In a small bowl, whisk together the fresh lemon juice, olive oil, salt, and pepper to make the dressing. Pour the dressing over the salad ingredients.

4. **Toss Gently:** Gently toss all the ingredients together until evenly coated with the dressing.

5. **Garnish and Serve:** Garnish with chopped fresh cilantro or parsley if desired. Serve the fenugreek and chickpea salad immediately as a light and nutritious dish.

Nutrition per Serving (Serves 4)

- **Calories:** 200 kcal
- **Protein:** 8 grams
- **Fat:** 8 grams
- **Carbohydrates:** 25 grams

- **Fiber:** 7 grams
- **Sugar:** 5 grams
- **Vitamin A:** 500 IU
- **Vitamin C:** 20 mg
- **Calcium:** 60 mg

This fenugreek and chickpea salad is not only flavorful but also packed with protein, fiber, and essential vitamins. It's a perfect salad option for those looking to add more plant-based protein and greens to their diet. Enjoy this light and nutritious dish as a refreshing meal or a side to complement any main course!

Recipe 28: Avocado and Chickpea Wrap

Easy and Filling Wrap

This Avocado and Chickpea Wrap is a delicious and satisfying meal that's quick to prepare and perfect for a healthy lunch or dinner option. Packed with creamy avocado, protein-rich chickpeas, and fresh vegetables, it's a balanced and flavorful wrap.

Ingredients

- 4 whole wheat tortilla wraps
- 1 ripe avocado, sliced
- 1 cup cooked chickpeas (canned or boiled)
- 1 cup mixed salad greens
- 1/2 cucumber, thinly sliced
- 1/4 cup red onion, thinly sliced
- 2 tablespoons hummus or tahini
- Fresh lemon juice, to taste
- Salt and pepper to taste

Instructions

1. **Prepare Ingredients:** If using canned chickpeas, rinse and drain them. If using dried chickpeas, cook according to package instructions until tender.

2. **Assemble Wraps:** Lay out the whole wheat tortilla wraps on a clean surface. Spread a tablespoon of hummus or tahini on each wrap.

3. **Layer Ingredients:** Divide the sliced avocado, cooked chickpeas, mixed salad greens, cucumber slices, and thinly sliced red onion evenly among the tortilla wraps.

4. **Season and Roll:** Squeeze fresh lemon juice over the fillings. Season with salt and pepper to taste. Roll up the wraps tightly, folding in the sides to enclose the fillings.

5. **Serve:** Cut each wrap in half diagonally. Serve immediately, or wrap tightly in foil or parchment paper for a portable meal.

Nutrition per Serving (Makes 4 wraps)

- **Calories:** 350 kcal
- **Protein:** 10 grams
- **Fat:** 12 grams
- **Carbohydrates:** 50 grams
- **Fiber:** 10 grams
- **Sugar:** 5 grams
- **Vitamin A:** 400 IU
- **Vitamin C:** 15 mg
- **Calcium:** 100 mg

These avocado and chickpea wraps are not only easy to make but also provide a good balance of protein, healthy fats, and fiber. Enjoy them as a nutritious and filling meal option for lunch or dinner!

Recipe 29: Avocado and Spinach Salad

Refreshing and Healthy Salad

This Avocado and Spinach Salad is a refreshing and nutritious dish that combines creamy avocado with fresh spinach leaves and a zesty dressing. It's simple to make, packed with vitamins and minerals, and perfect as a light meal or side salad.

Ingredients

- 200 grams fresh spinach leaves
- 1 ripe avocado, sliced
- 1/2 cup cherry tomatoes, halved
- 1/4 cup red onion, thinly sliced
- 1/4 cup cucumber, diced
- 2 tablespoons olive oil
- 1 tablespoon balsamic vinegar
- 1 teaspoon Dijon mustard
- Salt and pepper to taste
- Optional: toasted nuts or seeds for garnish

Instructions

1. **Prepare Salad Ingredients:** Wash and dry the fresh spinach leaves. Slice the avocado, halve the cherry tomatoes, thinly slice the red onion, and dice the cucumber.

2. **Assemble Salad:** In a large salad bowl, combine the fresh spinach leaves, sliced avocado, halved cherry tomatoes, thinly sliced red onion, and diced cucumber.

3. **Make Dressing:** In a small bowl, whisk together the olive oil, balsamic vinegar, Dijon mustard, salt, and pepper until well combined.

4. **Dress Salad:** Drizzle the dressing over the salad ingredients. Gently toss the salad until everything is evenly coated with the dressing.

5. **Garnish and Serve:** Optionally, sprinkle toasted nuts or seeds over the salad for added crunch and flavor. Serve the avocado and spinach salad immediately as a refreshing and healthy dish.

Nutrition per Serving (Serves 2)

- **Calories:** 250 kcal
- **Protein:** 5 grams
- **Fat:** 20 grams
- **Carbohydrates:** 15 grams
- **Fiber:** 8 grams
- **Sugar:** 5 grams
- **Vitamin A:** 6000 IU
- **Vitamin C:** 40 mg
- **Calcium:** 120 mg

This avocado and spinach salad is not only refreshing but also provides a good source of vitamins, minerals, and healthy fats. Enjoy it as a nutritious meal or a side salad to complement any main dish!

Recipe 30: Spicy Ginseng Tea

Energizing and Warming Drink

This Spicy Ginseng Tea is a revitalizing beverage that combines the energizing properties of ginseng with the warmth of spices. It's perfect for boosting energy levels and providing a comforting drink during colder days.

Ingredients

- 1 teaspoon ginseng powder or 2-3 ginseng tea bags
- 1 inch piece fresh ginger, sliced
- 2 cups water
- 1 cinnamon stick
- 2-3 whole cloves
- Honey or maple syrup, to taste (optional)
- Lemon slices for garnish (optional)

Instructions

1. **Prepare Ingredients:** In a small saucepan, combine the ginseng powder or ginseng tea bags, fresh ginger slices, cinnamon stick, whole cloves, and water.

2. **Simmer:** Bring the mixture to a boil over medium-high heat. Once boiling, reduce the heat to low and let it simmer for 10-15 minutes to infuse the flavors.

3. **Strain and Serve:** Remove the saucepan from heat and strain the tea into mugs to remove the solids. Discard the solids.

4. **Sweeten (optional):** Stir in honey or maple syrup to taste, if desired, for added sweetness.

5. **Garnish and Enjoy:** Garnish each mug with a slice of lemon, if using. Serve the spicy ginseng tea hot and enjoy its energizing and warming benefits.

Nutrition per Serving (Makes 2 servings)

- **Calories:** 10 kcal
- **Protein:** 0 grams
- **Fat:** 0 grams
- **Carbohydrates:** 2 grams
- **Fiber:** 0 grams
- **Sugar:** 0 grams

- **Vitamin C:** 0 mg
- **Iron:** 0 mg

This spicy ginseng tea is not only energizing but also comforting with its warming spices. Enjoy it as a revitalizing drink to boost your energy levels and provide a soothing experience.

CONCLUSION

In conclusion, maintaining men's sexual health through nutrition is closely tied to the consumption of a balanced diet rich in essential nutrients. By incorporating foods such as fruits like bananas and watermelon, nuts like almonds and walnuts, lean proteins such as salmon and chicken, whole grains like oats and quinoa, herbs and spices including garlic, ginseng, and fenugreek, healthy fats like olive oil and nuts, and indulging in dark chocolate and shellfish in moderation, individuals can promote their overall well-being.

Experimenting with the provided recipes can help individuals seamlessly incorporate these nutritious foods into their daily meals. Whether enjoying a quick Avocado and Chickpea Wrap for lunch, savoring a nutritious Avocado and Spinach Salad for dinner, or warming up with a comforting Spicy Ginseng Tea, each dish offers a delicious way to support optimal health.

Maintaining a healthy lifestyle extends beyond diet alone. Regular physical activity, adequate sleep, stress management, and avoiding harmful habits contribute to holistic well-being. By making informed choices and embracing a balanced approach to nutrition and lifestyle, men can enhance their vitality and overall quality of life.

Remember, small changes can lead to significant improvements in health over time. Start today by incorporating these healthy practices into your routine and enjoy the benefits of a vibrant and active life.